DIET COOKBOOK FOR CIRRHOSIS OF THE LIVER

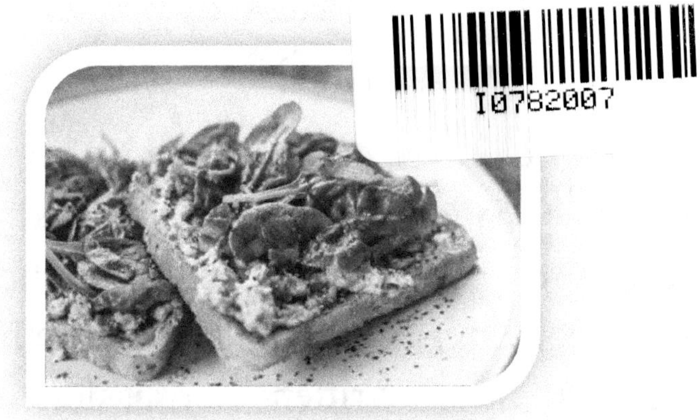

Natural plant based recipes to boost your renal function and support your liver cirrhosis

D.R CATHERINE THOMAS

TABLE OF CONTENT

INTRODUCTION

Life has a way of bringing us unexpected gifts, often in the most surprising places. It was during a nutrition conference in the picturesque city of Oslo, Norway, that I encountered one such gift a story of hope and healing that profoundly shaped my understanding of the power of nutrition.

As a seasoned nutritionist, I've spent years advocating for the importance of a balanced and wholesome diet. But it was during this conference that I reconnected with an old friend, Ingrid, whose journey with liver cirrhosis left an indelible mark on me.

Ingrid and I first met years ago at a seminar in New York, where our shared passion for nutrition and health sparked a lasting friendship. Over the years, we kept in touch sporadically, exchanging professional insights and personal updates. However, it wasn't until that fateful conference in Norway that I learned about the incredible transformation she had undergone.

Ingrid had been diagnosed with liver cirrhosis, a condition that had cast a shadow over her vibrant life. The prognosis was grim, and her doctors advised her to prepare for the worst. Yet, Ingrid was not one to surrender easily.

She immersed herself in research, seeking alternative ways to support her liver health beyond conventional medicine.

Her journey led her to discover the profound impact of diet on liver function and overall health. With determination and meticulous planning, Ingrid crafted a diet rich in anti-inflammatory foods, packed with nutrients that promoted healing and vitality. She embraced a lifestyle that not only nourished her body but also revitalized her spirit.

Over time, the results were nothing short of miraculous. Ingrid's liver function improved dramatically, and her symptoms diminished. Her doctors were astounded, calling her recovery a testament to the body's remarkable ability to heal when given the right tools. Ingrid's story became a beacon of hope for many, illustrating the transformative power of nutrition.

Inspired by Ingrid's journey, I felt compelled to share this knowledge with a broader audience. This cookbook, "Diet Cookbook for Cirrhosis of the Liver," is a culmination of years of research, professional experience, and heartfelt stories like Ingrid's. It is designed to be a guide for those seeking to combat liver cirrhosis through nutritious and flavorful anti-inflammatory recipes.

In the following pages, you'll find a variety of recipes that are not only delicious but also tailored to support liver health. These dishes are crafted to provide the essential nutrients needed to help manage liver cirrhosis naturally, enhancing your overall well-being.

Ingrid's story is a testament to the incredible resilience of the human spirit and the transformative power of the right diet. I hope this cookbook inspires you to embrace a journey of healing and vitality, just as Ingrid did. Here's to your health and happiness!

Warm regards,

Dr. Catherine Thomas

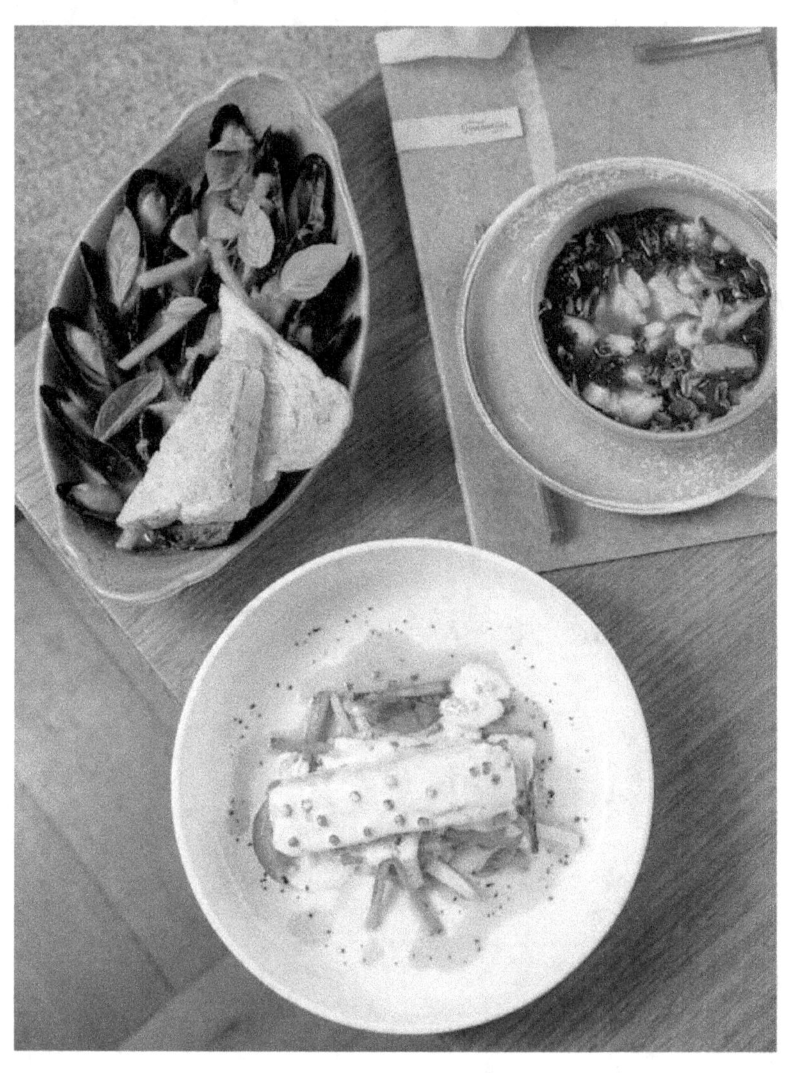

CHAPTER 1:

Understanding Cirrhosis of the Liver

Cirrhosis of the liver is a serious and potentially life-threatening condition characterized by the replacement of healthy liver tissue with scar tissue. This scarring disrupts the liver's ability to function properly, impairing its capacity to detoxify the blood, produce essential proteins, and regulate various metabolic processes. As the disease progresses, liver function deteriorates, leading to a cascade of health problems.

Types of Cirrhosis

Cirrhosis can be categorized into several types, each with distinct underlying causes:

1. **Alcoholic Cirrhosis:** Chronic and excessive alcohol consumption is a leading cause of cirrhosis. Over time, alcohol damages liver cells, leading to inflammation and scarring. This type of cirrhosis is often associated with a history of heavy drinking spanning many years.

2. **Non-Alcoholic Steatohepatitis (NASH):** NASH is a form of non-alcoholic fatty liver disease (NAFLD) that progresses to cirrhosis. It is characterized by fat accumulation in the liver, inflammation, and liver cell damage. Risk factors include obesity, diabetes, high cholesterol, and metabolic syndrome.

3. **Chronic Viral Hepatitis:** Hepatitis B and C infections are significant causes of cirrhosis globally. These viruses cause chronic liver inflammation, leading to progressive scarring over time.

4. **Biliary Cirrhosis:** This type results from long-term bile duct damage and inflammation, leading to bile build-up in the liver. Primary biliary cholangitis (PBC) and primary sclerosing cholangitis (PSC) are examples of conditions that can cause biliary cirrhosis.

5. **Genetic Disorders:** Certain inherited conditions, such as hemochromatosis (excessive iron accumulation) and Wilson's disease (excessive copper accumulation), can lead to liver cirrhosis.

6. **Autoimmune Hepatitis:** In this condition, the immune system mistakenly attacks liver cells, causing chronic inflammation and damage that can progress to cirrhosis.

The development of cirrhosis is typically a gradual process resulting from chronic liver damage. Key causes include:

Chronic Alcohol Abuse: Prolonged excessive drinking is one of the most common causes of cirrhosis. The liver metabolizes alcohol, producing toxic substances that can damage liver cells.

Chronic Hepatitis B and C: Persistent infection with these viruses causes ongoing liver inflammation, leading to scarring and cirrhosis over time.

Non-Alcoholic Fatty Liver Disease (NAFLD): Fat accumulation in the liver, often associated with obesity, diabetes, and metabolic syndrome, can lead to inflammation and cirrhosis.

Autoimmune Diseases: Conditions like autoimmune hepatitis cause the immune system to attack liver cells, leading to chronic inflammation and scarring.

Genetic Disorders: Inherited conditions that cause abnormal accumulation of substances in the liver, such as iron or copper, can lead to cirrhosis.

Biliary Diseases: Chronic bile duct diseases can cause bile build-up and liver damage, resulting in cirrhosis.

Cirrhosis often progresses silently, with symptoms becoming apparent only when liver damage is advanced. Common symptoms include:

Fatigue: A persistent feeling of tiredness and weakness.

Jaundice: Yellowing of the skin and eyes due to elevated bilirubin levels.

Edema: Swelling in the legs, ankles, and feet due to fluid retention.

Ascites: Accumulation of fluid in the abdomen, causing swelling and discomfort.

Bruising and Bleeding: Increased tendency to bruise or bleed easily due to impaired production of blood clotting factors.

Itchy Skin: Persistent itching, often due to bile salts deposited in the skin.

Spider Angiomas: Small, spider-like blood vessels visible under the skin.

Weight Loss: Unintentional weight loss and muscle wasting.

Confusion and Cognitive Changes: Hepatic encephalopathy can cause confusion, memory problems, and personality changes due to toxin buildup in the brain.

While cirrhosis can be a daunting diagnosis, there are several preventive measures that can significantly reduce the risk:

1. **Moderate Alcohol Consumption**: Limiting alcohol intake is crucial. For those with liver disease, complete abstinence is often recommended.

2. **Healthy Diet**: A balanced diet rich in fruits, vegetables, whole grains, lean proteins, and healthy fats can support liver health. Avoiding processed foods, sugary beverages, and high-fat meals is beneficial.

3. **Regular Exercise**: Maintaining a healthy weight through regular physical activity can prevent NAFLD and reduce the risk of cirrhosis.

4. **Vaccination**: Vaccination against hepatitis B can prevent infection and subsequent liver damage. Practicing safe behaviors to avoid hepatitis C transmission is also important.

5. **Routine Health Screenings**: Regular check-ups and liver function tests can help detect early signs of liver disease, allowing for timely intervention.

6. **Avoiding Toxins**: Limiting exposure to harmful chemicals and toxins can protect the liver from damage.

7. **Managing Chronic Conditions**: Proper management of conditions like diabetes, high cholesterol, and obesity can reduce the risk of cirrhosis.

8. **Medication Awareness**: Being cautious with medications, especially over-the-counter drugs and supplements that can harm the liver, is essential.

By understanding the types, causes, symptoms, and preventive measures associated with cirrhosis, individuals can take proactive steps to protect their liver health. Early intervention and lifestyle modifications can make a significant difference, offering hope for a healthier future.

Managing cirrhosis of the liver involves more than just medical treatments; it requires a carefully planned diet to support liver function and overall health. Following a liver-friendly diet can help reduce liver stress, prevent further damage, and alleviate symptoms. Here's a guide on how to follow a cirrhosis-friendly diet:

1. Limit Sodium Intake

Excessive sodium can lead to fluid retention and worsen edema and ascites, common complications of cirrhosis. Aim to consume no more than 1,500 to 2,000 milligrams of sodium per day. Here are some tips:

Avoid Processed Foods: Processed and packaged foods, including canned soups, deli meats, and frozen meals, often contain high sodium levels.

Read Labels: Check nutrition labels for sodium content. Choose low-sodium or no-salt-added options whenever possible.

Cook at Home: Preparing meals at home allows you to control the amount of salt used. Use herbs and spices to add flavor without salt.

2. Eat a Balanced Diet

A balanced diet provides the necessary nutrients to support liver health and overall well-being. Focus on:

Fruits and Vegetables: Aim for a variety of colorful fruits and vegetables. They are rich in vitamins, minerals, and antioxidants that support liver health.

Whole Grains: Choose whole grains like brown rice, quinoa, oats, and whole wheat bread. They provide fiber, which aids digestion and helps manage blood sugar levels.

Lean Proteins: Opt for lean protein sources such as poultry, fish, beans, and legumes. Protein is essential for tissue repair and immune function. However, if you have hepatic encephalopathy, your doctor may recommend adjusting your protein intake.

Healthy Fats: Include sources of healthy fats, such as avocados, nuts, seeds, and olive oil. These fats support cell function and provide energy without straining the liver.

3. Limit Fat Intake

A diet high in unhealthy fats can exacerbate liver damage and contribute to fatty liver disease. To limit fat intake:

Avoid Fried Foods: Choose baked, grilled, or steamed options instead of fried foods.

Select Low-Fat Dairy: Opt for low-fat or fat-free dairy products to reduce saturated fat intake.

Choose Lean Cuts: When eating meat, select lean cuts and trim visible fat.

4. Monitor Protein Intake

Protein needs can vary based on the severity of liver disease. Generally, moderate protein intake is recommended to prevent muscle wasting while avoiding excessive amounts that can lead to hepatic encephalopathy. Consult your healthcare provider to determine the appropriate protein level for your condition.

5. Stay Hydrated

Proper hydration is crucial for liver health and overall bodily functions. Drink plenty of water throughout the day. Limit sugary drinks, sodas, and alcohol, as they can worsen liver damage and dehydration.

6. Avoid Alcohol

Alcohol is a major cause of liver damage and should be completely avoided by those with cirrhosis. Even small amounts can exacerbate the condition and accelerate liver deterioration.

7. Vitamin and Mineral Supplements

Cirrhosis can lead to deficiencies in vitamins and minerals, such as vitamin D, calcium, and B vitamins. Your doctor may recommend supplements to ensure you meet your nutritional needs.

8. Frequent, Small Meals

Eating smaller, more frequent meals can help manage symptoms like nausea and improve nutrient absorption. Aim for five to six small meals throughout the day instead of three large ones.

By following these dietary guidelines, individuals with cirrhosis can help support their liver health, reduce complications, and improve their overall quality of life.

CHAPTER 2:

Core Benefits of Following a Cirrhosis of the Liver Diet

Following a cirrhosis-friendly diet is essential for managing the condition and promoting overall health. This diet is designed to reduce liver stress, support liver function, and prevent further damage. Here are the core benefits of adhering to such a diet:

1. Reduces Fluid Retention

One of the primary benefits of a cirrhosis diet is its ability to help manage fluid retention. Cirrhosis can cause complications like edema (swelling in the legs) and ascites (fluid accumulation in the abdomen). By limiting sodium intake, which is a core component of this diet, individuals can reduce the risk of fluid retention and associated complications.

2. Supports Liver Function

A balanced diet rich in essential nutrients supports liver function. The liver requires various vitamins and minerals to perform its detoxification, metabolism, and protein synthesis functions.

A cirrhosis diet ensures that the liver gets the necessary nutrients to operate efficiently and repair itself as much as possible.

3. Prevents Malnutrition

Cirrhosis can lead to malnutrition due to impaired nutrient absorption and metabolism. By following a diet that includes a variety of fruits, vegetables, whole grains, lean proteins, and healthy fats, individuals can maintain adequate nutrition levels. This helps in preserving muscle mass, maintaining energy levels, and supporting overall health.

4. Manages Hepatic Encephalopathy

Hepatic encephalopathy is a condition caused by the accumulation of toxins in the brain due to impaired liver function. By monitoring and adjusting protein intake, a cirrhosis diet can help manage the symptoms of hepatic encephalopathy. Consuming the right amount of protein is crucial to prevent the buildup of ammonia, which can exacerbate this condition.

5. Promotes Healthy Weight Management

Obesity and fatty liver disease can worsen cirrhosis. A cirrhosis diet emphasizes whole foods, lean proteins, and healthy fats, which can help individuals achieve and maintain a healthy weight.

Proper weight management reduces the strain on the liver and improves overall health outcomes.

6. Improves Digestive Health

High fiber intake from fruits, vegetables, and whole grains promotes healthy digestion and regular bowel movements. This is particularly important for individuals with cirrhosis, as it helps prevent constipation and reduces the risk of hepatic encephalopathy by promoting the excretion of toxins.

7. Reduces Inflammation

Anti-inflammatory foods, such as fruits, vegetables, nuts, seeds, and fatty fish, are staples of a cirrhosis diet. These foods help reduce liver inflammation and oxidative stress, which are key contributors to liver damage. Lowering inflammation can slow the progression of cirrhosis and improve liver function.

8. Enhances Immune Function

A diet rich in vitamins, minerals, and antioxidants supports the immune system. Individuals with cirrhosis are often at higher risk for infections due to compromised liver function. Strengthening the immune system through proper nutrition can help reduce the risk of infections and improve overall health.

9. Boosts Energy Levels

Malnutrition and liver dysfunction can lead to chronic fatigue in individuals with cirrhosis.

 A well-balanced diet ensures a steady supply of energy by providing complex carbohydrates, lean proteins, and healthy fats. This helps maintain energy levels and improve the quality of life.

10. Improves Mental Health

Good nutrition positively impacts mental health. By managing hepatic encephalopathy through diet and ensuring a steady intake of essential nutrients, individuals can experience improved cognitive function and mood. This contributes to a better overall sense of well-being and quality of life.

Following a cirrhosis-friendly diet is a powerful tool in managing the condition and enhancing overall health. By reducing fluid retention, supporting liver function, preventing malnutrition, managing hepatic encephalopathy, promoting healthy weight management, improving digestive health, reducing inflammation, enhancing immune function, boosting energy levels, and improving mental health, individuals can significantly improve their quality of life.

Here is a 7-day sample meal plan designed to support liver health and manage cirrhosis. Each day includes balanced meals with low sodium, lean proteins, whole grains, and plenty of fruits and vegetables.

Day 1

Breakfast

Oatmeal with fresh berries and a sprinkle of chia seeds

Herbal tea

Lunch

Grilled chicken breast with quinoa salad (mixed with chopped vegetables and olive oil)

Steamed broccoli

Snack

Apple slices with almond butter

Dinner

Baked salmon with lemon and dill

Brown rice

Steamed green beans

Day 2

Breakfast

Smoothie with spinach, banana, blueberries, and unsweetened almond milk

Whole grain toast

Lunch

Turkey and avocado wrap in a whole wheat tortilla

Carrot sticks

Snack

Greek yogurt with honey and walnuts

Dinner

Stir-fried tofu with mixed vegetables (broccoli, bell peppers, carrots) and low-sodium soy sauce

Brown rice

Breakfast

Scrambled eggs with spinach and tomatoes

Whole grain toast

Lunch

Lentil soup with mixed vegetables

Side salad with mixed greens, cherry tomatoes, and olive oil dressing

Snack

Sliced cucumbers and hummus

Dinner

Baked chicken thighs with rosemary and garlic

Quinoa

Steamed asparagus

Day 4

Breakfast

Greek yogurt parfait with granola and fresh fruit

Herbal tea

Lunch

Tuna salad (with olive oil, lemon juice, and herbs) on a bed of mixed greens

Whole grain crackers

Snack

Orange slices

Dinner

Grilled shrimp with whole wheat pasta and a tomato basil sauce

Steamed zucchini

Day 5

Breakfast

Whole grain waffles with fresh strawberries and a drizzle of maple syrup

Herbal tea

Lunch

Chickpea and vegetable stir-fry

Brown rice

Snack

Pear slices with a handful of walnuts

Dinner

Baked cod with lemon and herbs

Mashed sweet potatoes

Steamed spinach

Day 6

Breakfast

Smoothie bowl with blended mango, spinach, and unsweetened almond milk, topped with granola and coconut flakes

Herbal tea

Lunch

Turkey and vegetable quinoa bowl (mixed with bell peppers, cucumbers, and olive oil)

Side of steamed broccoli

Snack

Baby carrots with guacamole

Dinner

Grilled chicken and vegetable kebabs

Whole grain couscous

Roasted Brussels sprouts

Breakfast

Whole grain oatmeal with sliced banana and a sprinkle of flaxseeds

Herbal tea

Lunch

Spinach and feta stuffed bell peppers

Side salad with mixed greens and a light vinaigrette

Snack

Handful of almonds and dried cranberries

Dinner

Baked trout with garlic and lemon

Quinoa

Steamed mixed vegetables (carrots, green beans, and cauliflower)

This meal plan emphasizes low sodium, lean proteins, healthy fats, and plenty of fruits and vegetables to support liver health.

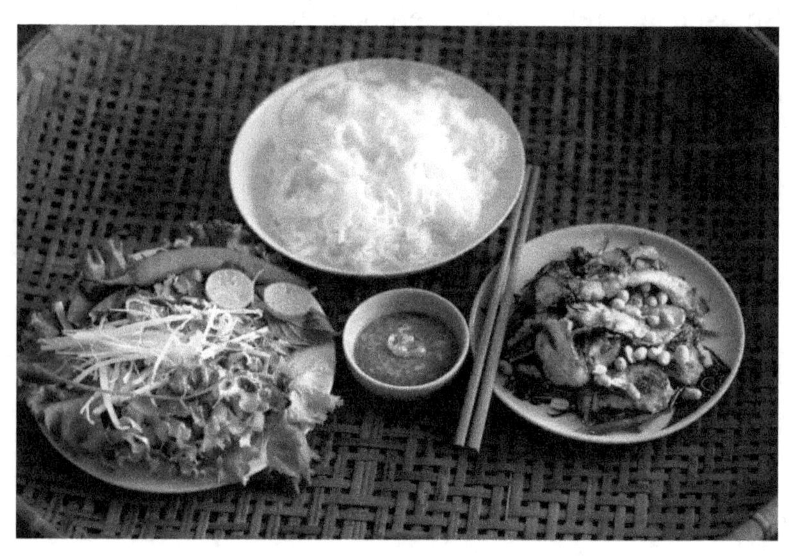

CHAPTER 3:

BREAKFAST RECIPES:

❖ Berry Oatmeal

Ingredients:

1 cup rolled oats

2 cups water

1/2 cup fresh blueberries

1/2 cup fresh strawberries, sliced

1 tbsp chia seeds

1 tbsp honey (optional)

Preparation:

1. In a pot, bring water to a boil.

2. Add oats and reduce to a simmer. Cook for 5 minutes, stirring occasionally.

3. Stir in berries and chia seeds. Cook for another 2 minutes.

4. Drizzle with honey if desired.

Cooking Time: 10 minutes

Nutritional Value (per serving): Calories: 250, Protein: 6g, Carbohydrates: 45g, Fat: 5g, Fiber: 8g

❖ Spinach and Tomato Scramble

Ingredients:

2 large eggs

1/2 cup fresh spinach, chopped

1/2 cup cherry tomatoes, halved

1 tbsp olive oil

Salt and pepper to taste

Preparation:

1. Heat olive oil in a pan over medium heat.

2. Add spinach and tomatoes, cook for 2-3 minutes.

3. Beat eggs and pour into the pan. Stir until scrambled and cooked through, about 3-4 minutes.

4. Season with salt and pepper.

Cooking Time: 10 minutes

Nutritional Value (per serving): Calories: 200, Protein: 14g, Carbohydrates: 6g, Fat: 14g, Fiber: 2g

❖ Greek Yogurt Parfait

Ingredients:

1 cup Greek yogurt

1/2 cup granola

1/2 cup mixed berries (blueberries, raspberries)

1 tbsp honey

Preparation:

1. In a bowl, layer Greek yogurt, granola, and berries.

2. Drizzle with honey.

Cooking Time: 5 minutes

Nutritional Value (per serving): Calories: 300, Protein: 15g, Carbohydrates: 45g, Fat: 10g, Fiber: 5g

❖ Avocado Toast

Ingredients:

1 slice whole grain bread, toasted

1/2 ripe avocado, mashed

1 tbsp lemon juice

Salt and pepper to taste

Preparation:

1. Toast the bread.

2. Mash avocado with lemon juice, salt, and pepper.

3. Spread avocado mixture on toast.

Cooking Time: 5 minutes

Nutritional Value (per serving): Calories: 220, Protein: 5g, Carbohydrates: 30g, Fat: 10g, Fiber: 7g

❖ Smoothie Bowl

Ingredients:

1 cup spinach

1 banana

1/2 cup frozen mango

1/2 cup unsweetened almond milk

1 tbsp chia seeds

1 tbsp granola

Preparation:

1. Blend spinach, banana, mango, and almond milk until smooth.

2. Pour into a bowl and top with chia seeds and granola.

Cooking Time: 5 minutes

Nutritional Value (per serving): Calories: 250, Protein: 5g, Carbohydrates: 50g, Fat: 7g, Fiber: 8g

❖ Quinoa Breakfast Bowl

Ingredients:

1/2 cup cooked quinoa

1/4 cup fresh blueberries

1/4 cup fresh raspberries

1 tbsp chopped almonds

1 tbsp honey

Preparation:

1. Combine quinoa, blueberries, raspberries, and almonds in a bowl.

2. Drizzle with honey.

Cooking Time: 5 minutes (using pre-cooked quinoa)
Nutritional Value (per serving): Calories: 270, Protein: 7g, Carbohydrates: 50g, Fat: 7g, Fiber: 8g

❖ Apple Cinnamon Overnight Oats

Ingredients:

1/2 cup rolled oats

1/2 cup unsweetened almond milk

1/4 cup unsweetened applesauce

1/4 tsp cinnamon

1 tbsp chia seeds

Preparation:

1. Combine all ingredients in a jar.

2. Refrigerate overnight.

Cooking Time: 5 minutes (plus overnight refrigeration) **Nutritional Value (per serving):** Calories: 220, Protein: 6g, Carbohydrates: 40g, Fat: 5g, Fiber: 7g

❖ Banana Nut Smoothie

Ingredients:

1 banana

1/2 cup unsweetened almond milk

1 tbsp almond butter

1 tbsp chia seeds

1/4 tsp vanilla extract

Preparation:

1. Blend all ingredients until smooth.

Cooking Time: 5 minutes

Nutritional Value (per serving): Calories: 250, Protein: 5g, Carbohydrates: 40g, Fat: 10g, Fiber: 6g

❖ Whole Grain Waffles

Ingredients:

1 cup whole grain waffle mix

1/2 cup water

1/4 cup fresh strawberries, sliced

- 1 tbsp pure maple syrup

Preparation:

1. Mix waffle batter according to package instructions.

2. Cook in a waffle maker until golden brown.

3. Top with strawberries and drizzle with maple syrup.

Cooking Time: 10 minutes

Nutritional Value (per serving): Calories: 250, Protein: 6g, Carbohydrates: 45g, Fat: 6g, Fiber: 5g

❖ Chia Pudding

Ingredients:

1/4 cup chia seeds

1 cup unsweetened almond milk

1 tbsp honey

1/2 cup mixed berries

Preparation:

1. Mix chia seeds, almond milk, and honey in a jar.

2. Refrigerate for at least 4 hours or overnight.

3. Top with mixed berries before serving.

Cooking Time: 5 minutes

(plus refrigeration time) **Nutritional Value (per serving):** Calories: 300, Protein: 8g, Carbohydrates: 40g, Fat: 15g, Fiber: 15g

Lunch:

❖ **Quinoa and Vegetable Salad**

Ingredients:

1 cup cooked quinoa

1/2 cup cherry tomatoes, halved

1/2 cucumber, diced

1/4 cup red bell pepper, diced

2 tbsp olive oil

1 tbsp lemon juice

Salt and pepper to taste

Preparation:

1. In a large bowl, combine quinoa, cherry tomatoes, cucumber, and bell pepper.

2. In a small bowl, whisk together olive oil, lemon juice, salt, and pepper.

3. Pour the dressing over the salad and toss to combine.

Cooking Time: 10 minutes

(using pre-cooked quinoa) **Nutritional Value (per serving):** Calories: 300, Protein: 8g, Carbohydrates: 35g, Fat: 15g, Fiber: 5g

❖ Grilled Chicken and Avocado Wrap

Ingredients:

1 whole wheat tortilla

1 grilled chicken breast, sliced

1/2 avocado, sliced

1/2 cup mixed greens

1 tbsp hummus

Preparation:

1. Spread hummus on the tortilla.

2. Add sliced chicken, avocado, and mixed greens.

3. Roll up the tortilla and cut in half.

Cooking Time: 10 minutes (using pre-cooked chicken)

 Nutritional Value (per serving): Calories: 350, Protein: 25g, Carbohydrates: 30g, Fat: 15g, Fiber: 8g

❖ Lentil Soup

Ingredients:

1 cup dried lentils

1 onion, chopped

2 carrots, chopped

2 celery stalks, chopped

4 cups low-sodium vegetable broth

1 tbsp olive oil

1 tsp cumin

1/2 tsp turmeric

Preparation:

1. In a large pot, heat olive oil over medium heat.

2. Add onion, carrots, and celery; cook for 5 minutes.

3. Stir in lentils, cumin, turmeric, and vegetable broth.

4. Bring to a boil, then reduce heat and simmer for 25-30 minutes, until lentils are tender.

Cooking Time: 40 minutes

Nutritional Value (per serving): Calories: 250, Protein: 15g, Carbohydrates: 40g, Fat: 5g, Fiber: 15g

❖ Turkey and Spinach Stuffed Peppers

Ingredients:

2 bell peppers, halved and seeded

1 cup cooked ground turkey

1 cup cooked quinoa

1/2 cup spinach, chopped

1/2 cup diced tomatoes

1 tsp Italian seasoning

Preparation:

1. Preheat oven to 375°F (190°C).

2. In a bowl, mix ground turkey, quinoa, spinach, tomatoes, and Italian seasoning.

3. Stuff bell pepper halves with the mixture.

4. Place in a baking dish and bake for 20-25 minutes.

Cooking Time: 30 minutes

Nutritional Value (per serving): Calories: 300, Protein: 25g, Carbohydrates: 35g, Fat: 8g, Fiber: 7g

❖ Chickpea and Vegetable Stir-Fry

Ingredients:

1 can (15 oz) chickpeas, drained and rinsed

1 cup broccoli florets

1 red bell pepper, sliced

1 zucchini, sliced

2 tbsp olive oil

2 tbsp low-sodium soy sauce

1 tsp garlic powder

Preparation:

1. Heat olive oil in a large pan over medium-high heat.

2. Add broccoli, bell pepper, and zucchini; cook for 5 minutes.

3. Add chickpeas, soy sauce, and garlic powder; cook for another 5 minutes, stirring frequently.

Cooking Time: 15 minutes

Nutritional Value (per serving): Calories: 300, Protein: 10g, Carbohydrates: 40g, Fat: 12g, Fiber: 10g

❖ Baked Salmon with Asparagus

Ingredients:

1 salmon fillet (about 6 oz)

1 cup asparagus spears

1 tbsp olive oil

1 lemon, sliced

Salt and pepper to taste

Preparation:

1. Preheat oven to 400°F (200°C).

2. Place salmon and asparagus on a baking sheet.

3. Drizzle with olive oil and season with salt and pepper.

4. Top with lemon slices.

5. Bake for 15-20 minutes, until salmon is cooked through.

Cooking Time: 20 minutes

Nutritional Value (per serving): Calories: 350, Protein: 30g, Carbohydrates: 8g, Fat: 22g, Fiber: 4g

❖ Chicken and Vegetable Quinoa Bowl

Ingredients:

1 cup cooked quinoa

1 grilled chicken breast, sliced

1/2 cup cherry tomatoes, halved

1/2 cup cucumber, diced

1/4 cup feta cheese, crumbled

2 tbsp olive oil

1 tbsp balsamic vinegar

Preparation:

1. In a bowl, combine quinoa, chicken, cherry tomatoes, cucumber, and feta cheese.

2. In a small bowl, whisk together olive oil and balsamic vinegar.

3. Pour dressing over the bowl and toss to combine.

Cooking Time: 10 minutes (using pre-cooked chicken and quinoa)

Nutritional Value (per serving): Calories: 400, Protein: 30g, Carbohydrates: 40g, Fat: 18g, Fiber: 6g

❖ Vegetable and Hummus Wrap

Ingredients:

1 whole wheat tortilla

1/4 cup hummus

1/4 cup shredded carrots

1/4 cup cucumber, sliced

1/4 cup red bell pepper, sliced

1/4 cup mixed greens

Preparation:

1. Spread hummus on the tortilla.

2. Add shredded carrots, cucumber, bell pepper, and mixed greens.

3. Roll up the tortilla and cut in half.

Cooking Time: 5 minutes

Nutritional Value (per serving): Calories: 250, Protein: 8g, Carbohydrates: 35g, Fat: 10g, Fiber: 8g

❖ Spinach and Feta Stuffed Chicken Breast

Ingredients:

1 chicken breast, butterflied

1/2 cup fresh spinach, chopped

1/4 cup feta cheese, crumbled

1 tbsp olive oil

Salt and pepper to taste

Preparation:

1. Preheat oven to 375°F (190°C).

2. In a bowl, mix spinach and feta cheese.

3. Stuff the chicken breast with the spinach mixture and secure with toothpicks.

4. Heat olive oil in an oven-safe pan over medium heat and sear the chicken for 2-3 minutes on each side.

5. Transfer the pan to the oven and bake for 20 minutes.

Cooking Time: 25 minutes

Nutritional Value (per serving): Calories: 300, Protein: 35g, Carbohydrates: 2g, Fat: 18g, Fiber: 1g

❖ Turkey and Avocado Salad

Ingredients:

2 cups mixed greens

1/2 cup cooked turkey breast, sliced

1/2 avocado, sliced

1/4 cup cherry tomatoes, halved

1 tbsp olive oil

1 tbsp lemon juice

Salt and pepper to taste

Preparation:

1. In a bowl, combine mixed greens, turkey, avocado, and cherry tomatoes.

2. In a small bowl, whisk together olive oil, lemon juice, salt, and pepper.

3. Drizzle dressing over the salad and toss to combine.

Cooking Time: 10 minutes (using pre-cooked turkey)

Nutritional Value (per serving): Calories: 300, Protein: 25g, Carbohydrates: 12g, Fat: 18g, Fiber: 6g

❖ Grilled Salmon with Steamed Broccoli

Ingredients:

1 salmon fillet (about 6 oz)

1 tbsp olive oil

1 lemon, sliced

Salt and pepper to taste

1 cup broccoli florets

Preparation:

1. Preheat grill to medium-high heat.

2. Brush salmon with olive oil and season with salt and pepper.

3. Grill salmon for 4-5 minutes on each side, until cooked through.

4. Steam broccoli in a pot for 5-7 minutes.

5. Serve salmon with lemon slices and steamed broccoli.

Cooking Time: 15 minutes

Nutritional Value (per serving): Calories: 350, Protein: 30g, Carbohydrates: 8g, Fat: 22g, Fiber: 4g

❖ Chicken and Vegetable Stir-Fry

Ingredients:

1 chicken breast, sliced

1 cup broccoli florets

1 red bell pepper, sliced

1 carrot, sliced

2 tbsp olive oil

2 tbsp low-sodium soy sauce

1 tsp garlic powder

Preparation:

1. Heat olive oil in a large pan over medium-high heat.

2. Add chicken and cook for 5-7 minutes, until browned.

3. Add broccoli, bell pepper, and carrot; cook for another 5 minutes.

4. Stir in soy sauce and garlic powder; cook for 2 more minutes.

Cooking Time: 15 minutes

Nutritional Value (per serving): Calories: 300, Protein: 25g, Carbohydrates: 20g, Fat: 12g, Fiber: 6g

❖ Quinoa Stuffed Bell Peppers

Ingredients:

2 bell peppers, halved and seeded

1 cup cooked quinoa

1/2 cup black beans, drained and rinsed

1/2 cup corn kernels

1/4 cup diced tomatoes

1 tsp cumin

1 tsp chili powder

Preparation:

1. Preheat oven to 375°F (190°C).

2. In a bowl, mix quinoa, black beans, corn, tomatoes, cumin, and chili powder.

3. Stuff bell pepper halves with the mixture.

4. Place in a baking dish and bake for 20-25 minutes.

Cooking Time: 30 minutes

Nutritional Value (per serving): Calories: 300, Protein: 10g, Carbohydrates: 50g, Fat: 5g, Fiber: 10g

❖ Baked Cod with Asparagus

Ingredients:

1 cod fillet (about 6 oz)

1 tbsp olive oil

1 lemon, sliced

1 cup asparagus spears

Salt and pepper to taste

Preparation:

1. Preheat oven to 400°F (200°C).

2. Place cod and asparagus on a baking sheet.

3. Drizzle with olive oil and season with salt and pepper.

4. Top with lemon slices.

5. Bake for 15-20 minutes, until cod is cooked through.

Cooking Time: 20 minutes

Nutritional Value (per serving): Calories: 250, Protein: 30g, Carbohydrates: 10g, Fat: 10g, Fiber: 4g

❖ Turkey and Spinach Meatballs

Ingredients:

1 lb ground turkey

1 cup fresh spinach, chopped

1/4 cup whole wheat breadcrumbs

1 egg

1 tsp Italian seasoning

1/2 tsp garlic powder

Salt and pepper to taste

Preparation:

1. Preheat oven to 375°F (190°C).

2. In a bowl, mix ground turkey, spinach, breadcrumbs, egg, Italian seasoning, garlic powder, salt, and pepper.

3. Form into meatballs and place on a baking sheet.

4. Bake for 20-25 minutes, until cooked through.

Cooking Time: 25 minutes

Nutritional Value (per serving): Calories: 250, Protein: 30g, Carbohydrates: 10g, Fat: 10g, Fiber: 2g

❖ Vegetable Lentil Stew

Ingredients:

1 cup dried lentils

1 onion, chopped

2 carrots, chopped

2 celery stalks, chopped

4 cups low-sodium vegetable broth

1 tbsp olive oil

1 tsp cumin

1/2 tsp turmeric

Preparation:

1. In a large pot, heat olive oil over medium heat.

2. Add onion, carrots, and celery; cook for 5 minutes.

3. Stir in lentils, cumin, turmeric, and vegetable broth.

4. Bring to a boil, then reduce heat and simmer for 25-30 minutes, until lentils are tender.

Cooking Time: 40 minutes

Nutritional Value (per serving): Calories: 250, Protein: 15g, Carbohydrates: 40g, Fat: 5g, Fiber: 15g

❖ Zucchini Noodles with Pesto

Ingredients:

2 zucchinis, spiralized

1/4 cup pesto

1 tbsp olive oil

1/4 cup cherry tomatoes, halved

Preparation:

1. Heat olive oil in a pan over medium heat.

2. Add zucchini noodles and cook for 2-3 minutes.

3. Stir in pesto and cherry tomatoes; cook for another 2 minutes.

Cooking Time: 10 minutes

Nutritional Value (per serving): Calories: 200, Protein: 5g, Carbohydrates: 10g, Fat: 18g, Fiber: 4g

❖ Baked Chicken with Sweet Potatoes

Ingredients:

1 chicken breast

1 sweet potato, diced

1 tbsp olive oil

1 tsp paprika

Salt and pepper to taste

Preparation:

1. Preheat oven to 375°F (190°C).

2. Place chicken and sweet potatoes on a baking sheet.

3. Drizzle with olive oil and season with paprika, salt, and pepper.

4. Bake for 25-30 minutes, until chicken is cooked through and sweet potatoes are tender.

Cooking Time: 30 minutes

Nutritional Value (per serving): Calories: 350, Protein: 30g, Carbohydrates: 30g, Fat: 10g, Fiber: 6g

❖ Shrimp and Vegetable Skewers

Ingredients:

1/2 lb shrimp, peeled and deveined

1 red bell pepper, chopped

1 zucchini, sliced

1 tbsp olive oil

1 lemon, juiced

Salt and pepper to taste

Preparation:

1. Preheat grill to medium-high heat.

2. Thread shrimp, bell pepper, and zucchini onto skewers.

3. Brush with olive oil and lemon juice; season with salt and pepper.

4. Grill for 2-3 minutes on each side, until shrimp is opaque and vegetables are tender.

Cooking Time: 10 minutes

Nutritional Value (per serving): Calories: 200, Protein: 25g, Carbohydrates: 10g, Fat: 7g, Fiber: 3g

❖ Spaghetti Squash with Marinara Sauce

Ingredients:

1 spaghetti squash

2 cups marinara sauce

1 tbsp olive oil

1/4 cup Parmesan cheese, grated

Salt and pepper to taste

Preparation:

1. Preheat oven to 375°F (190°C).

2. Cut spaghetti squash in half and remove seeds.

3. Drizzle with olive oil and season with salt and pepper.

4. Place cut side down on a baking sheet and bake for 35-40 minutes.

5. Scrape out the squash strands with a fork.

6. Heat marinara sauce in a pot over medium heat.

7. Serve spaghetti squash topped with marinara sauce and Parmesan cheese.

Cooking Time: 40 minutes

Nutritional Value (per serving): Calories: 250, Protein: 7g, Carbohydrates: 40g, Fat: 10g, Fiber: 8g

Desserts and Snacks:

❖ Greek Yogurt with Berries

Ingredients:

1 cup Greek yogurt

1/2 cup mixed berries (strawberries, blueberries, raspberries)

1 tbsp honey

Preparation:

1. In a bowl, combine Greek yogurt and honey.

2. Top with mixed berries.

Cooking Time: 5 minutes

Nutritional Value (per serving): Calories: 150, Protein: 15g, Carbohydrates: 20g, Fat: 2g, Fiber: 4g

❖ Apple Slices with Almond Butter

Ingredients:

1 apple, sliced

2 tbsp almond butter

Preparation:

1. Core and slice the apple.

2. Serve apple slices with almond butter for dipping.

Cooking Time: 5 minutes

Nutritional Value (per serving): Calories: 200, Protein: 4g, Carbohydrates: 28g, Fat: 10g, Fiber: 5g

❖ Chia Seed Pudding

Ingredients:

1/4 cup chia seeds

1 cup almond milk

1 tbsp honey

1/2 tsp vanilla extract

Preparation:

1. In a bowl, mix chia seeds, almond milk, honey, and vanilla extract.

2. Refrigerate for at least 4 hours or overnight until it thickens.

Cooking Time: **5 minutes (plus refrigeration)**

Nutritional Value (per serving): Calories: 180, Protein: 5g, Carbohydrates: 20g, Fat: 9g, Fiber: 10g

❖ Oatmeal Energy Balls

Ingredients:

1 cup rolled oats

1/2 cup almond butter

1/4 cup honey

1/4 cup dark chocolate chips

Preparation:

1. In a bowl, combine rolled oats, almond butter, honey, and chocolate chips.

2. Roll into small balls and refrigerate for 30 minutes.

Cooking Time: 10 minutes (plus refrigeration)

Nutritional Value (per serving): Calories: 100 (per ball), Protein: 3g, Carbohydrates: 12g, Fat: 5g, Fiber: 2g

❖ Baked Apple Chips

Ingredients:

2 apples, thinly sliced

1 tsp cinnamon

Preparation:

1. Preheat oven to 225°F (110°C).

2. Arrange apple slices on a baking sheet lined with parchment paper.

3. Sprinkle with cinnamon.

4. Bake for 1.5-2 hours, flipping halfway through, until crisp.

Cooking Time: 2 hours   Nutritional Value (per serving): Calories: 80, Protein: 0g, Carbohydrates: 22g, Fat: 0g, Fiber: 4g

Ingredients:

1 cucumber, sliced

1/2 cup hummus

Preparation:

1. Slice the cucumber into rounds.

2. Top each cucumber slice with a dollop of hummus.

Cooking Time: 5 minutes

Nutritional Value (per serving): Calories: 100, Protein: 4g, Carbohydrates: 12g, Fat: 5g, Fiber: 3g

❖ Frozen Banana Bites

Ingredients:

2 bananas, sliced

1/4 cup dark chocolate chips, melted

1 tbsp shredded coconut

Preparation:

1. Slice bananas and arrange on a baking sheet lined with parchment paper.

2. Drizzle melted dark chocolate over banana slices.

3. Sprinkle with shredded coconut.

4. Freeze for at least 1 hour.

Cooking Time: 5 minutes (plus freezing)

Nutritional Value (per serving): Calories: 150, Protein: 2g, Carbohydrates: 30g, Fat: 5g, Fiber: 3g

❖ Avocado Chocolate Mousse

Ingredients:

1 ripe avocado

2 tbsp cocoa powder

2 tbsp honey

1/4 cup almond milk

Preparation:

1. In a blender, combine avocado, cocoa powder, honey, and almond milk.

2. Blend until smooth and creamy.

3. Chill in the refrigerator for 30 minutes before serving.

Cooking Time: 5 minutes (plus refrigeration)

Nutritional Value (per serving): Calories: 200, Protein: 3g, Carbohydrates: 22g, Fat: 14g, Fiber: 7g

❖ Cottage Cheese and Pineapple

Ingredients:

1 cup low-fat cottage cheese

1/2 cup pineapple chunks (fresh or canned in juice)

Preparation:

1. In a bowl, combine cottage cheese and pineapple chunks.

Cooking Time: 5 minutes

Nutritional Value (per serving): Calories: 180, Protein: 15g, Carbohydrates: 20g, Fat: 5g, Fiber: 1g

❖ Berry Smoothie

Ingredients:

1/2 cup blueberries

1/2 cup strawberries

1/2 cup Greek yogurt

1 cup almond milk

1 tbsp honey

Preparation:

1. In a blender, combine blueberries, strawberries, Greek yogurt, almond milk, and honey.

2. Blend until smooth.

Cooking Time: 5 minutes

Nutritional Value (per serving): Calories: 200, Protein: 8g, Carbohydrates: 35g, Fat: 5g, Fiber: 5g

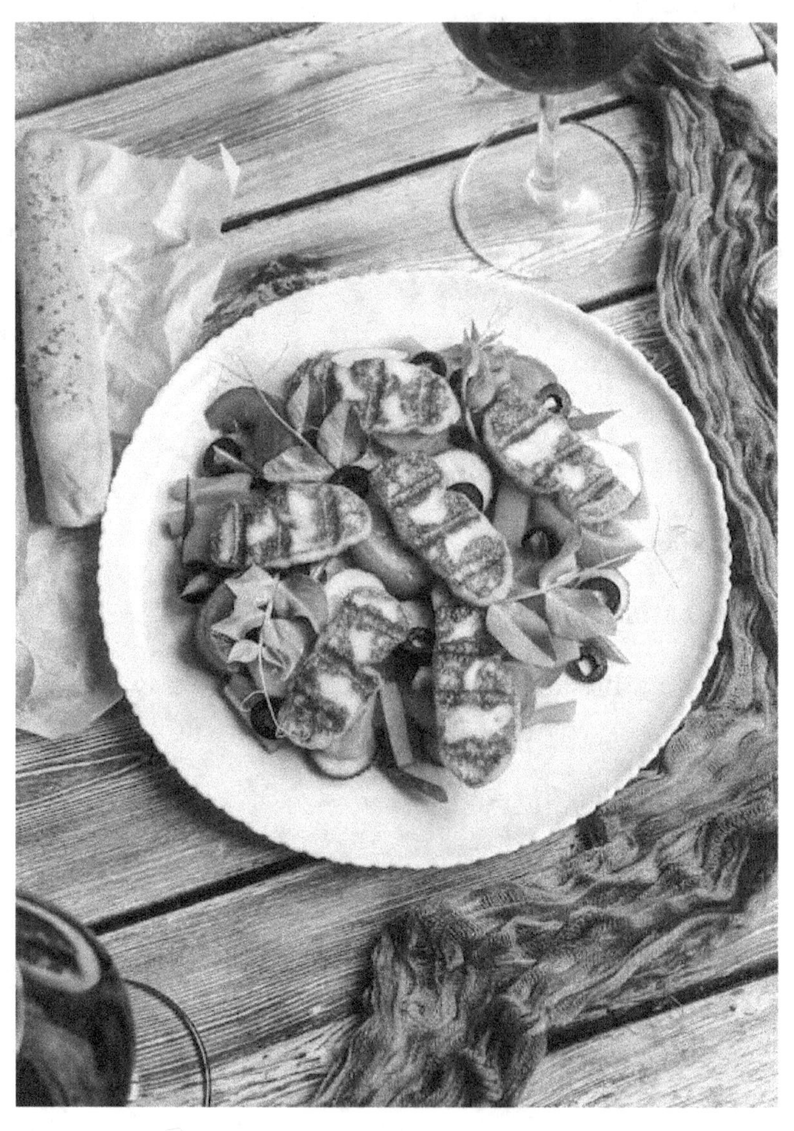

CONCLUSION

Cirrhosis of the liver is a complex condition that demands careful attention to diet and lifestyle. This cookbook has provided you with a wealth of nutritious, delicious, and easy-to-prepare recipes specifically designed to support liver health. Each recipe is crafted to offer the nutrients your body needs while avoiding ingredients that can exacerbate liver issues. By incorporating these meals into your daily routine, you can help manage cirrhosis more effectively and improve your overall well-being.

From wholesome breakfasts to satisfying dinners, along with tasty snacks and desserts, this cookbook offers a diverse range of options to keep your meals interesting and enjoyable. The emphasis on fresh vegetables, lean proteins, whole grains, and healthy fats ensures that you receive a balanced intake of essential nutrients. Moreover, these recipes are rich in anti-inflammatory ingredients that can help reduce liver inflammation and promote healing.

Adopting a liver-friendly diet is not just about managing a condition; it's about embracing a lifestyle that supports your long-term health. By making mindful food choices, you can significantly impact your liver function and quality of life.

This cookbook is more than a collection of recipes; it's a guide to living a healthier, more vibrant life.

As you embark on this journey, remember that every small change you make can lead to significant improvements. Be patient with yourself, and celebrate each step forward. The transition to a new way of eating might feel challenging at first, but the benefits are well worth the effort. You have the power to positively influence your health and well-being through the foods you choose.

Let this cookbook be your companion and inspiration. Embrace the delicious possibilities that a liver-friendly diet offers. By nourishing your body with the right foods, you are taking a proactive step towards a healthier future. Stay motivated, stay committed, and most importantly, enjoy the journey to better health

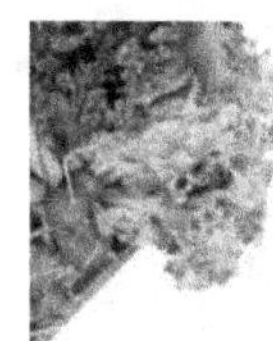

WEEKLY MEAL PLANNER

MONDAY	BREAKFAST	
	LUNCH	
	DINNER	
TUESDAY	BREAKFAST	
	LUNCH	
	DINNER	
WEDNESDAY	BREAKFAST	
	LUNCH	
	DINNER	
THURSDAY	BREAKFAST	
	LUNCH	
	DINNER	
FRIDAY	BREAKFAST	
	LUNCH	
	DINNER	
SARTURDAY	BREAKFAST	
	LUNCH	
	DINNER	
SUNDAY	BREAKFAST	
	LUNCH	
	DINNER	

GROCERY LIST

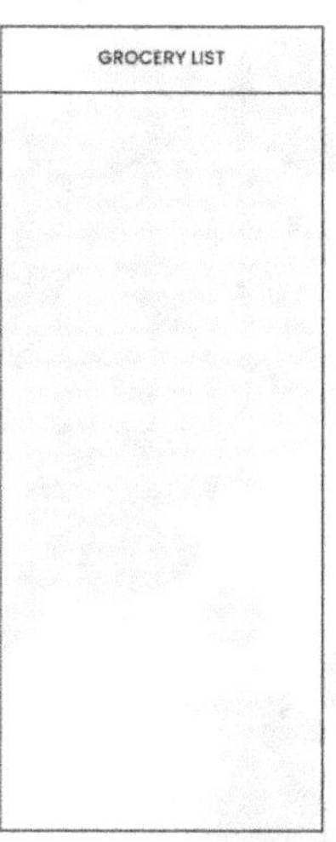

SNACKS

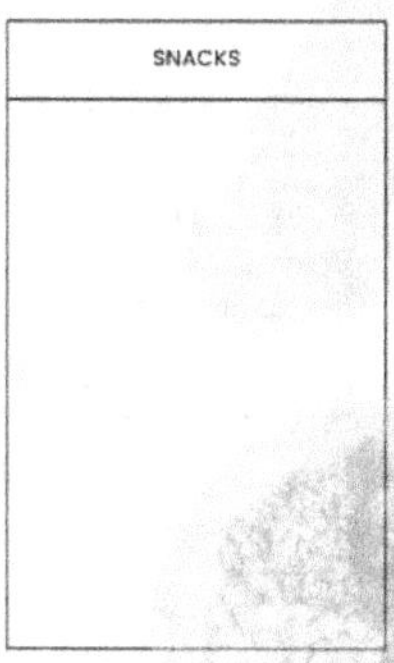

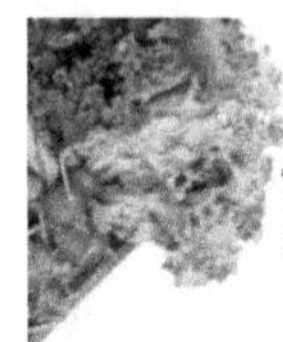

WEEKLY MEAL PLANNER

				GROCERY LIST
MONDAY	BREAKFAST			
	LUNCH			
	DINNER			
TUESDAY	BREAKFAST			
	LUNCH			
	DINNER			
WEDNESDAY	BREAKFAST			
	LUNCH			
	DINNER			
THURSDAY	BREAKFAST			
	LUNCH			
	DINNER			
FRIDAY	BREAKFAST			SNACKS
	LUNCH			
	DINNER			
SARTURDAY	BREAKFAST			
	LUNCH			
	DINNER			
SUNDAY	BREAKFAST			
	LUNCH			
	DINNER			

WEEKLY MEAL PLANNER

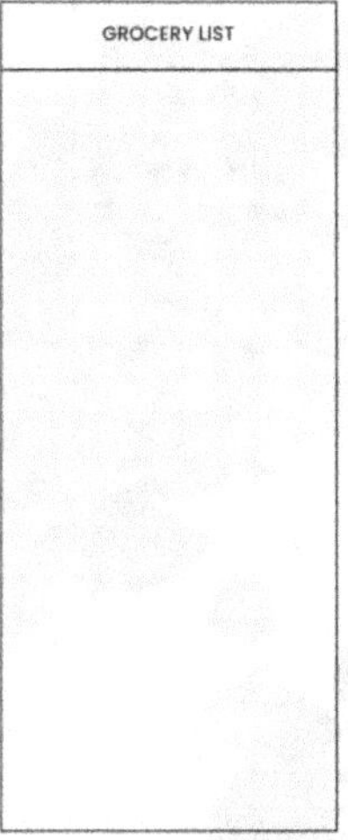

MONDAY	BREAKFAST	
	LUNCH	
	DINNER	
TUESDAY	BREAKFAST	
	LUNCH	
	DINNER	
WEDNESDAY	BREAKFAST	
	LUNCH	
	DINNER	
THURSDAY	BREAKFAST	
	LUNCH	
	DINNER	
FRIDAY	BREAKFAST	
	LUNCH	
	DINNER	
SARTURDAY	BREAKFAST	
	LUNCH	
	DINNER	
SUNDAY	BREAKFAST	
	LUNCH	
	DINNER	

GROCERY LIST

SNACKS

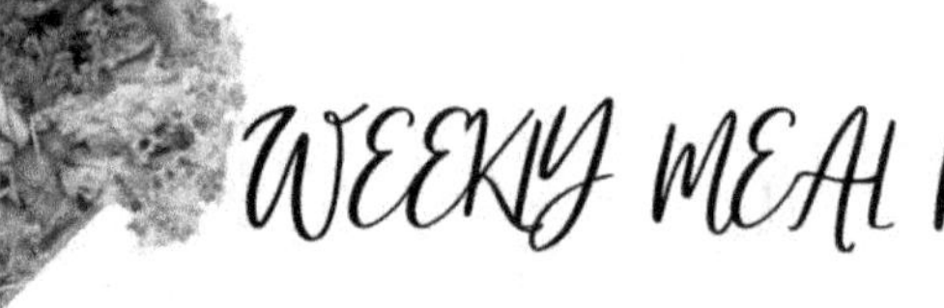

WEEKLY MEAL PLANNER

			GROCERY LIST
MONDAY	BREAKFAST		
	LUNCH		
	DINNER		
TUESDAY	BREAKFAST		
	LUNCH		
	DINNER		
WEDNESDAY	BREAKFAST		
	LUNCH		
	DINNER		
THURSDAY	BREAKFAST		
	LUNCH		
	DINNER		
FRIDAY	BREAKFAST		SNACKS
	LUNCH		
	DINNER		
SARTURDAY	BREAKFAST		
	LUNCH		
	DINNER		
SUNDAY	BREAKFAST		
	LUNCH		
	DINNER		

WEEKLY MEAL PLANNER

MONDAY	BREAKFAST	
	LUNCH	
	DINNER	
TUESDAY	BREAKFAST	
	LUNCH	
	DINNER	
WEDNESDAY	BREAKFAST	
	LUNCH	
	DINNER	
THURSDAY	BREAKFAST	
	LUNCH	
	DINNER	
FRIDAY	BREAKFAST	
	LUNCH	
	DINNER	
SARTURDAY	BREAKFAST	
	LUNCH	
	DINNER	
SUNDAY	BREAKFAST	
	LUNCH	
	DINNER	

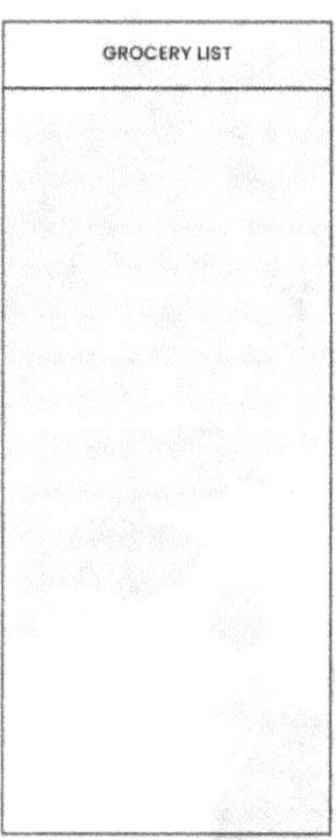

GROCERY LIST

SNACKS

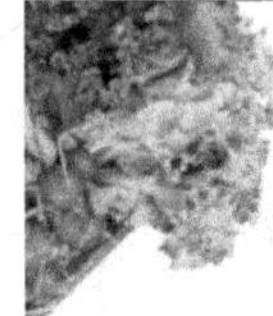

WEEKLY MEAL PLANNER

			GROCERY LIST
MONDAY	BREAKFAST		
	LUNCH		
	DINNER		
TUESDAY	BREAKFAST		
	LUNCH		
	DINNER		
WEDNESDAY	BREAKFAST		
	LUNCH		
	DINNER		
THURSDAY	BREAKFAST		
	LUNCH		
	DINNER		
FRIDAY	BREAKFAST		SNACKS
	LUNCH		
	DINNER		
SARTURDAY	BREAKFAST		
	LUNCH		
	DINNER		
SUNDAY	BREAKFAST		
	LUNCH		
	DINNER		

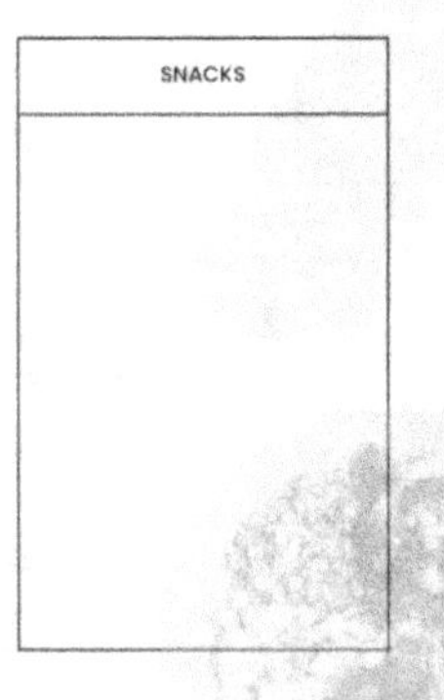

WEEKLY MEAL PLANNER

MONDAY	BREAKFAST	
	LUNCH	
	DINNER	
TUESDAY	BREAKFAST	
	LUNCH	
	DINNER	
WEDNESDAY	BREAKFAST	
	LUNCH	
	DINNER	
THURSDAY	BREAKFAST	
	LUNCH	
	DINNER	
FRIDAY	BREAKFAST	
	LUNCH	
	DINNER	
SARTURDAY	BREAKFAST	
	LUNCH	
	DINNER	
SUNDAY	BREAKFAST	
	LUNCH	
	DINNER	

GROCERY LIST

SNACKS

WEEKLY MEAL PLANNER

			GROCERY LIST
MONDAY	BREAKFAST		
	LUNCH		
	DINNER		
TUESDAY	BREAKFAST		
	LUNCH		
	DINNER		
WEDNESDAY	BREAKFAST		
	LUNCH		
	DINNER		
THURSDAY	BREAKFAST		
	LUNCH		
	DINNER		
FRIDAY	BREAKFAST		
	LUNCH		SNACKS
	DINNER		
SARTURDAY	BREAKFAST		
	LUNCH		
	DINNER		
SUNDAY	BREAKFAST		
	LUNCH		
	DINNER		

WEEKLY MEAL PLANNER

MONDAY	BREAKFAST	
	LUNCH	
	DINNER	
TUESDAY	BREAKFAST	
	LUNCH	
	DINNER	
WEDNESDAY	BREAKFAST	
	LUNCH	
	DINNER	
THURSDAY	BREAKFAST	
	LUNCH	
	DINNER	
FRIDAY	BREAKFAST	
	LUNCH	
	DINNER	
SARTURDAY	BREAKFAST	
	LUNCH	
	DINNER	
SUNDAY	BREAKFAST	
	LUNCH	
	DINNER	

GROCERY LIST

SNACKS

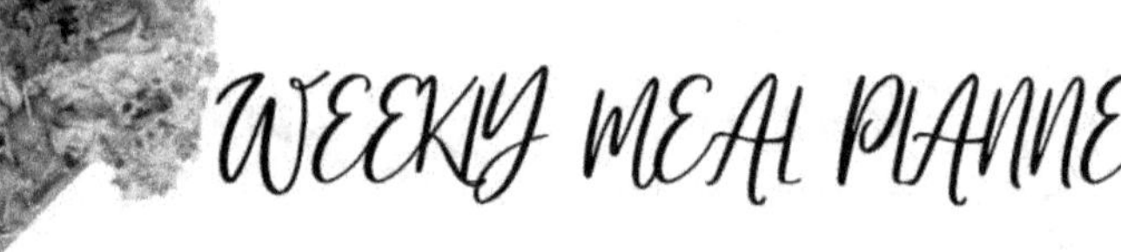

WEEKLY MEAL PLANNER

MONDAY	BREAKFAST	
	LUNCH	
	DINNER	
TUESDAY	BREAKFAST	
	LUNCH	
	DINNER	
WEDNESDAY	BREAKFAST	
	LUNCH	
	DINNER	
THURSDAY	BREAKFAST	
	LUNCH	
	DINNER	
FRIDAY	BREAKFAST	
	LUNCH	
	DINNER	
SARTURDAY	BREAKFAST	
	LUNCH	
	DINNER	
SUNDAY	BREAKFAST	
	LUNCH	
	DINNER	

GROCERY LIST

SNACKS

WEEKLY MEAL PLANNER

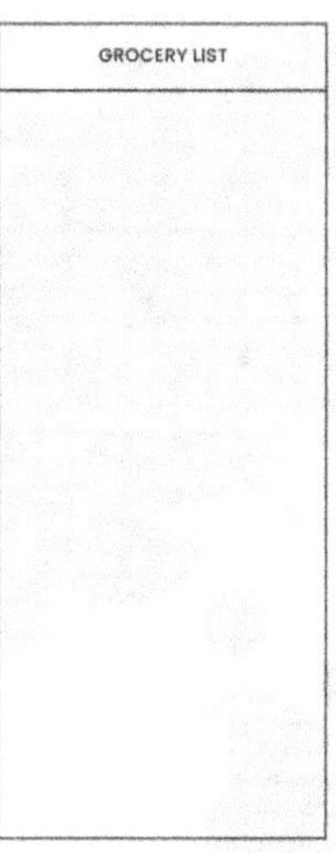

MONDAY	BREAKFAST	
	LUNCH	
	DINNER	
TUESDAY	BREAKFAST	
	LUNCH	
	DINNER	
WEDNESDAY	BREAKFAST	
	LUNCH	
	DINNER	
THURSDAY	BREAKFAST	
	LUNCH	
	DINNER	
FRIDAY	BREAKFAST	
	LUNCH	
	DINNER	
SARTURDAY	BREAKFAST	
	LUNCH	
	DINNER	
SUNDAY	BREAKFAST	
	LUNCH	
	DINNER	

GROCERY LIST

SNACKS

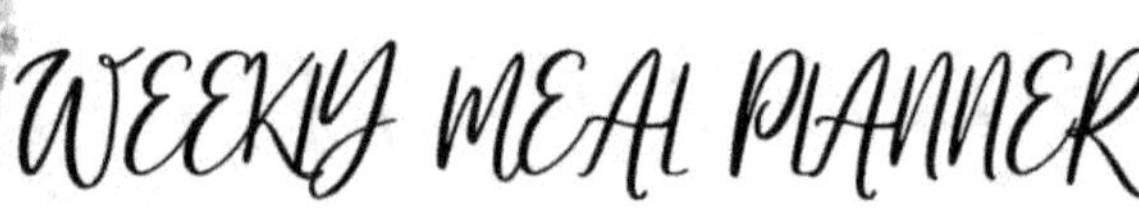

WEEKLY MEAL PLANNER

			GROCERY LIST
MONDAY — BREAKFAST			
MONDAY — LUNCH			
MONDAY — DINNER			
TUESDAY — BREAKFAST			
TUESDAY — LUNCH			
TUESDAY — DINNER			
WEDNESDAY — BREAKFAST			
WEDNESDAY — LUNCH			
WEDNESDAY — DINNER			
THURSDAY — BREAKFAST			
THURSDAY — LUNCH			
THURSDAY — DINNER			
FRIDAY — BREAKFAST			SNACKS
FRIDAY — LUNCH			
FRIDAY — DINNER			
SARTURDAY — BREAKFAST			
SARTURDAY — LUNCH			
SARTURDAY — DINNER			
SUNDAY — BREAKFAST			
SUNDAY — LUNCH			
SUNDAY — DINNER			

WEEKIY MEAL PLANNER

MONDAY	BREAKFAST	
	LUNCH	
	DINNER	
TUESDAY	BREAKFAST	
	LUNCH	
	DINNER	
WEDNESDAY	BREAKFAST	
	LUNCH	
	DINNER	
THURSDAY	BREAKFAST	
	LUNCH	
	DINNER	
FRIDAY	BREAKFAST	
	LUNCH	
	DINNER	
SARTURDAY	BREAKFAST	
	LUNCH	
	DINNER	
SUNDAY	BREAKFAST	
	LUNCH	
	DINNER	

GROCERY LIST

SNACKS

WEEKLY MEAL PLANNER

MONDAY	BREAKFAST	
	LUNCH	
	DINNER	
TUESDAY	BREAKFAST	
	LUNCH	
	DINNER	
WEDNESDAY	BREAKFAST	
	LUNCH	
	DINNER	
THURSDAY	BREAKFAST	
	LUNCH	
	DINNER	
FRIDAY	BREAKFAST	
	LUNCH	
	DINNER	
SARTURDAY	BREAKFAST	
	LUNCH	
	DINNER	
SUNDAY	BREAKFAST	
	LUNCH	
	DINNER	

GROCERY LIST

SNACKS